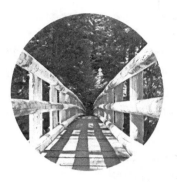

This Journal belongs to:

_____

_____

_____

_____

Advance Reader Comments

"White's eye for the details of everyday life shows that all of our existence is a miracle. Allow On LIFE to speak to you, and you will be richly rewarded."

– Larry Dossey, MD, Author: *One Mind: How Our Individual Mind Is Part of a Greater Consciousness and Why It Matters*

"This is just the book we need to help us get through a difficult time. Dr. White offers us hope when we need it the most."

– Mark C. Taylor, Columbia University, Author: *Seeing Silence*

"Reading On LIFE felt much like observing a flowing river on a summer day. The river is the same and yet different every moment."

– Praveen Suthrum, Entrepreneur, Author: *Scope Forward*

"Love this! Dr. White is a masterful teacher."

– Robyn Benson, Doctor of Oriental Medicine, Author: *Travel with Vitality: 7 Solutions for Sleeping Well, Staying Fit and Avoiding Illness*

"Welcome to my life! Dr. White gracefully helps us to be comfortable in periods of change."

– P. David Poling, PhD, Author: *Sea of Glory: A Novel*

"A cardiologist addresses the important things in life – from the heart. Recommended reading for many of my patients!"

– Mimi Guarneri, MD, Author: *108 Pearls to Awaken Your Healing Potential*

"Create new direction on your journey with Dr. White's perfect life prescription."

– Sunil Pai, MD, Author: *An Inflammation Nation*

"On LIFE - An essential, and may I say existential guidebook for living a life well lived!"

– Steven Gundry, MD, Author: *The Plant Paradox*

On LIFE JOURNAL

A Companion Workbook

Harvey J. White, MD

Guiding Conscious Living

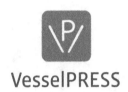

VesselPRESS

100601 4th Street NW
Albuquerque, NM 87114
www.VesselPressPublishing.com
505-828-3000

Copyright © 2020 by Harvey J. White MD

First Paperback Edition: July 2020
Library of Congress Control Number: 2020907647
- ISBN's -
Journal: 978-1-7348967-1-8
Book: 978-1-7348967-0-1
Mobi: 978-1-7348967-2-5
Epub: 978-1-7348967-3-2

Cover and Interior Design by Diane Rigoli, www.RigoliCreative.com
Photography by Kip Malone

Table of Contents

Make a DIFFERENCE

Plan to make a difference today
    See the goal
    Not just another day
    Not the easy way
    Stand for something
Be bold, aim high, have spirit
Make a difference today
                – HJW

Preface

Navigating life's waters can be fraught with shoals, tides, and headwinds. The astute ship's captain learns by observing and documenting the events of the voyage in the ship's log, providing a true-to-life record of those challenges and how they were over-come. Before GPS and satellite weather maps, the logs of those who had come before were priceless, allowing all sailors to become better at sea.

We all can learn something from those of an earlier generation, whether in their writing, storytelling, or simple observations. And yet real learning occurs when we assimilate such information for ourselves, developing our own opinions and working to apply them.

Both the sea captain and those of us who are on our own personal voyages must move beyond the theoretical. We must put what we have learned into practice. To do so requires that we eventually move from opinion to action.

The transition from theory to practice requires an important step: identifying and clarifying what we would do in a certain circumstance. Little works better than documenting our own personal plan. How would I manage a particular challenge? What would I do in a certain circumstance?

Writing down our plan in a journal can assist in this process.

This workbook-style journal, a companion piece to my book, On LIFE, provides such a platform. Read on and engage in the process to chart your course to a better life. Move on from land to adventures on the high seas!

A successful life: never easy, but forever possible.

Harvey J. White, MD
Albuquerque
January 2020

Introduction

Books about living in the challenging world that surrounds us can be addictive. Reading the words of another person can invigorate us. The author may set forth new ideas, articulate complex concepts, and identify energizing goals that in the moment stimulate the reader.

And yet reading is a passive endeavor. Often those lofty ideas and resounding principles are never put to practical use. An author's thoughts can be fleeting at best because the reader is immersed in the real world—one of distraction and immediacy. The book On LIFE, which serves as the foundation of this journal, is no exception. Certainly it identifies some of life's core challenges, along with guidelines for responding proactively to them. Binding its chapters together is the concept that we all are empowered to deal with life no matter what confronts us.

Ultimately the challenge for all of us is to become our own guides, to have our own philosophies and recipes for managing our life.

This journal-based workbook is designed to facilitate this process. It is not meant to provide pat answers but to help us find our own answers.

Laid out in chapters that mirror the companion book, the journal encourages the reader to recount personal stories, create unique observations and affirmations, and author their own individual advice. Often evoking remote memories, both positive and painful, this exercise is meant to serve like a flight simulator that puts pilots into virtual real-world flight challenges to help them develop reflexive responses to deal with them. Keying off these provocative questions, readers are encouraged to become even more engaged by developing their own particular thoughts on how to deal with a specific situation or challenge. Although On LIFE offers some ideas, the goal is for each of us to come up with our own solutions. These will survive when they're our own—self-generated, near indelible, readily retrieved, and ready for the moment.

Finally, nothing works better than a short catchphrase to orient ourselves to an optimal way of being. Noting some of the phrases which introduce and conclude the chapters in On LIFE, feel free to create your own—memorable for you and perhaps worthy of sharing with others.

Sail on!

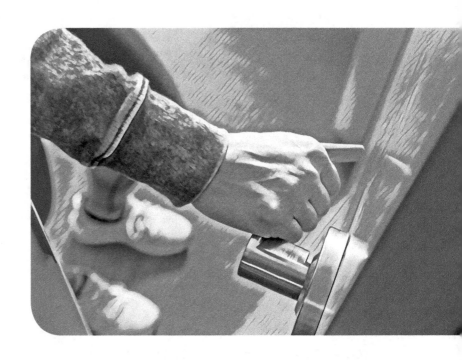

On BEGINNING

I Am in the Game

Beginnings can feel monumental. Starting an article for a magazine. Breaking ground on a new building. That first day at college. Often the decision to start something new can feel overwhelming. If we're viewing a beginning with fear or anxiety, how can we shift our mindset so it becomes a desired adventure? A look at your past may provide some answers.

MY STORY: At one time in my life I lived by the ocean and became a windsurfer. Yes, one of those crazy guys who flies around on the water on a board with a sail. Beginning such a complex and challenging sport was not natural for me. Thinking back, I remember that beginning, and I am so impressed by the sensations it created—freshness, renewal, commitment, feeling alive! Yes, I had many a wild adventure harnessing the wind, but it is the beginning I will never forget.

YOUR STORY (a memorable **BEGINNING**):

_____

_____

_____

_____

_____

_____

_____

_____

REFLECTIONS:

Observation 1. Why did you pick that moment in your life?

_____

_____

Observation 2. What emotions come to mind?

_____

_____

Observation 3. Did your worst fears come to pass? If so, how did you deal with the situation? If not, what did you learn from this particular beginning?

_____

_____

AFFIRMATIONS:

Commitment 1. The next time I prepare to start something new, I will. . .

_____

_____

Commitment 2. If I find myself struggling to begin something new, I will tell myself.

_____

_____

Commitment 3. I will choose a fresh start. I will be adventurous and try a new beginning that. . .

_____

_____

YOUR ADVICE (to revisit when you're struggling to begin something new):

_____

_____

_____

_____

_____

ROOM TO GROW:

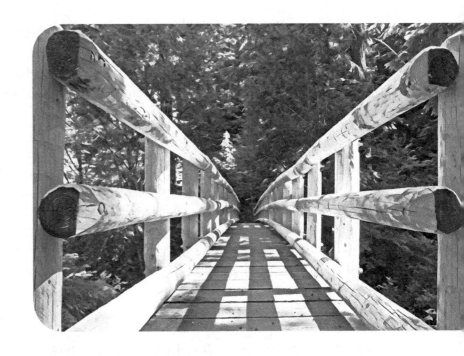

On CHANGE

All Will Be OK

Change is unsettling. Whether by choice or not, change interrupts our life's patterns, interferes with commitments, and creates subtle, and sometimes not so subtle stress. How we respond to change, however, determines whether the stresses are positive and constructive or negative and erosive. Pause and think about how you can manage change to make it an optimistic experience.

MY STORY: Academic medicine has its rewards, but I knew it wasn't for me. Three years on the faculty of an Ivy League school on the East Coast had proven that the future would not be clear sailing. Yet leaving the comfort of the familiar proved challenging. I searched and searched for a new professional environment. Finally, without a secure destination, I turned in my resignation. It took a bold move to get me to finally change.

YOUR STORY (choose a life **CHANGE** that stands out):

_____

_____

_____

_____

_____

_____

_____

_____

_____

REFLECTIONS:

Observation 1. Why did you choose this memorable life change?

_____

_____

Observation 2. Did you plan for this change or did it "happen" to you?

_____

_____

Observation 3. Would you go through it again? Why or why not? In either case, what did you learn about yourself?

_____

_____

AFFIRMATIONS:

Commitment 1. I will approach change with a fresh attitude of. . .

_____

_____

Commitment 2. If in doubt about a change, I will...

_____

_____

Commitment 3. If I waken at night worrying, I will...

_____

_____

YOUR ADVICE (to revisit when you're struggling with change):

_____

_____

_____

_____

_____

ROOM TO GROW:

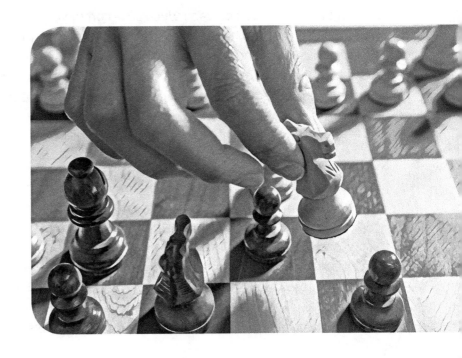

On DECISION

Have No Regrets

For many, making a decision can induce stress on the border of panic. Procrastination ensues, perhaps evolving to mental paralysis—until the decision is made for them! Having tools to move through challenging or even simple decisions can ease the process and minimize our potential for self-defeat. We need to be aware of our circumstances, make an informed decision to take action based on those circumstances, and accept the results, which are rarely irreversible.

MY STORY: A pioneering career in cardiology permitted me to live on the frontier of health care. Novel procedures, stimulating conferences, creative business structures, and even the founding of a new specialty hospital. My career's momentum came to a halt when the hospital I part-owned had to be sold due to new government regulations. What to do? Take the safe route and become an employed physician (the path of most aging doctors)? The decision to stake a claim in a new business at age 60 with the purpose of helping people prevent cardiovascular illness did not come easily. In the end, I knew my personal mission needed to become manifest. Vessel Health was created. As hard as this path has been, I have no regrets.

YOUR STORY (a challenging **DECISION**):

_____

_____

_____

_____

_____

_____

_____

_____

REFLECTIONS:

Observation 1. What stands out about that decision?

_____

_____

Observation 2. What was it that tipped the scales?

_____

_____

Observation 3. What did you learn from the experience? (Do you have any regrets? Would you make the same decision again?)

_____

_____

AFFIRMATIONS:

Commitment 1. When I encounter a difficult decision in the future, I will. . .

_____

_____

Commitment 2. To avoid procrastination, I will. . .

_____

_____

Commitment 3. When confronted with equally good or equally bad choices, I will. . .

_____

_____

YOUR ADVICE (to revisit when you find yourself mired in decision paralysis):

_____

_____

_____

_____

_____

ROOM TO GROW:

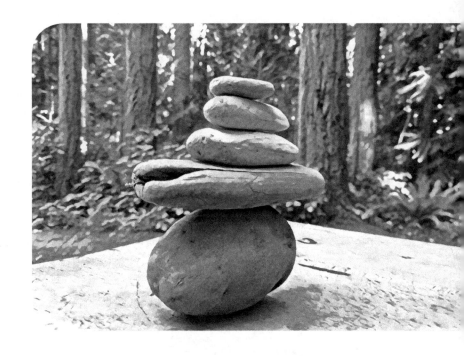

On GREATNESS

Reach For It

Being great is only for great people: Tiger Woods, Barack Obama, Robert Kennedy, Sandra Day O'Connor. Really? Are any of these notables preordained to be great? And do we have to accomplish great things to be great? It would seem that to be great, others must think we are. And yet, being great is a personal decision to strive for. It is in relationship only to ourselves—an attitude that fuels engagement and application to our own life.

MY STORY: As a highly engaged cardiologist, I often attend national conferences. Over the years they have morphed in content. Now, like the cable news networks, they rely on pundits to opine on a myriad of topics. A row of experts perched in front of the audience, extolling their opinions on this and that. They are the greats. Really? I return home to the front lines of health care, dealing with sick and worried patients daily. I choose to be great at that.

YOUR STORY (what will you be **GREAT** at?):

_____

_____

_____

_____

_____

_____

_____

_____

REFLECTIONS:

Observation 1. Are there times you feel inferior to those around you? If so, why do you think that is? What attitudes can remedy that?

_____

_____

Observation 2. Do you have fans, even if it is family, who think you are amazing? Do you agree with them? What can you strive for that will make you see yourself as amazing, or perhaps even more amazing than you are now?

_____

_____

Observation 3. How would aspiring to greatness make you feel empowered?

_____

_____

AFFIRMATIONS:

Commitment 1. One thing I am great at is...

_____

_____

Commitment 2. I will work toward being great at...

_____

_____

Commitment 3. I see myself as great just because I am me and because I...

_____

_____

YOUR ADVICE (to revisit when you feel greatness is beyond you):

_____

_____

_____

_____

_____

ROOM TO GROW:

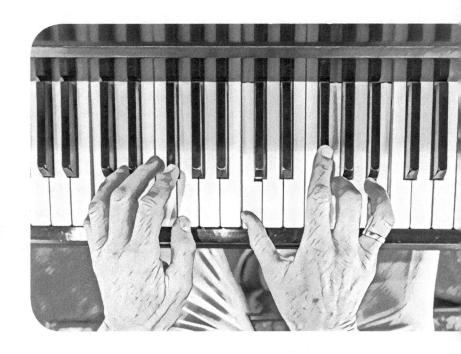

On CREATIVITY

Be Inspired

We are blessed with an amazing imagination. Our minds have permitted the development of remarkable organizations, religions, and technologies, as well as accomplishments in art and literature. But imagination and the power to create is not simply for social good but resides primarily in personal quests. We each have the capacity to create and express ourselves by generating something new. The rewards are remarkable.

MY STORY: As a child I was constantly building—model airplanes, scooters, go-carts, forts—and designing—rockets, other worlds. Later on, art—random sculpture. Even later, buildings—homes and hospitals. Now I find myself creating more in the abstract—businesses and ideas. But I miss the visual expression. For my upcoming college reunion I was asked what I would like to accomplish in the next ten years. Weld a sculpture!

YOUR STORY (what would you like to **CREATE**?):

_____

_____

_____

_____

_____

_____

_____

_____

REFLECTIONS:

Observation 1. What things did you create or what stories did you make up as a child?

_____

_____

Observation 2. When you put your attention and energy on something new, how does it feel?

_____

_____

Observation 3. Do you get the sense that as you have aged your creativity has waned? If so, what can you do to reignite that creative spark, keeping in mind the many ways to apply your creativity?

_____

_____

AFFIRMATIONS:

Commitment 1. I will cook the following new dish this weekend:

_____

_____

Commitment 2. I will spend more time looking at art with the goal of...

_____

_____

Commitment 3. I will express myself more creatively by. . .

_____

_____

YOUR ADVICE (to revisit when you forget how creative you can be):

_____

_____

_____

_____

_____

ROOM TO GROW:

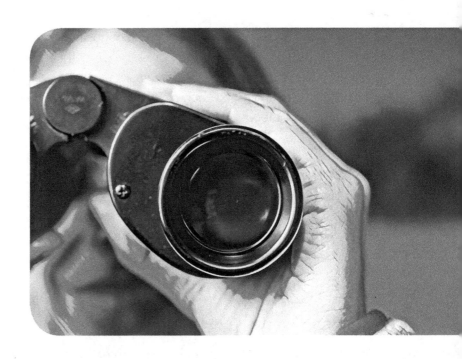

On FOCUS

Tune In

Our lives speed by at an enormous pace. Seconds become minutes, minutes become hours, days turn into years, and soon a life is complete. How do we ensure that we have maximized the experience? Through focus—that capacity to see things clearly and to experience and enjoy each moment. Without goals, our days are random. Goals intensify our focus.

MY STORY: My father, brother, and I planned an anniversary camping trip—thirty years since our first in the American West. We packed the truck and headed to southern Utah. Now twenty-five years later I remember so much in granular detail. Our route driven, campsites chosen, hikes taken, and vistas absorbed. I was totally alive. Today is Wednesday. What did I do last Wednesday? Good question.

YOUR STORY (recall an experience when everything was in **FOCUS**):

_____

_____

_____

_____

_____

_____

_____

_____

_____

REFLECTIONS:

Observation 1. What are the characteristics of your experience that seem most vivid?

_____

_____

Observation 2. How do you feel when you multitask or go through routines with a lack of focus?

_____

_____

Observation 3. What have you discovered that helps you focus and have mental clarity and improved memory? (For example, perhaps setting goals or photographing special moments helps you be more focused.)

_____

_____

AFFIRMATIONS:

Commitment 1. To enhance my focus, I will. . .

_____

_____

Commitment 2. The next time I go on a trip, I will. . .

_____

_____

Commitment 3. I will approach routines differently by. . .

_____

_____

YOUR ADVICE (to revisit when you find your days becoming just a blur):

_____

_____

_____

_____

_____

ROOM TO GROW:

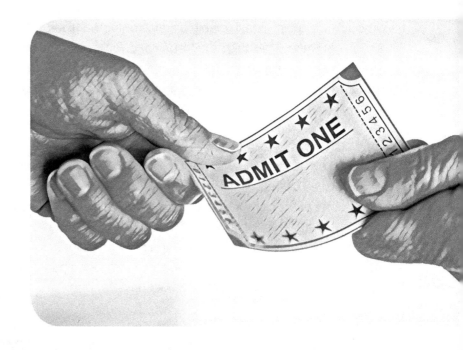

On CIRCUMSTANCE

See the Opportunity

Although we spend considerable time planning our lives, much of our experience is random. Someone drops by the house or calls you on the phone unexpectedly. Or you have an uncanny encounter at a party. Embedded in circumstance is considerable opportunity. How we view those experiences and grasp the moment, or even design our own circumstances to reach our goals, can enrich our lives.

MY STORY: We now have a brew pub down the street from our home. At first we gave it an occasional try when out-of-town family and friends came to visit. Recently, having a free Tuesday evening, I decided to take the experience one step further—sitting alone at the bar for dinner. To my amazement the house was packed. But it was easy to strike up a conversation with two guys sitting to my right. We shared a lot, including sports, a touch of politics, and how our careers have evolved. The long and short of it is that both fellows have become engaged participants in our preventive cardiovascular health clinic. Who would have thought?

YOUR STORY (describe an unexpected beneficial **CIRCUMSTANCE**):

_____

_____

_____

_____

_____

_____

_____

_____

REFLECTIONS:

Observation 1. Do you enjoy meeting new people? If not, why is it difficult? What was it about those circumstances, even if difficult, that may have benefited you?

_____

_____

Observation 2. When you are at a party or other social event, what can you do to take advantage of the opportunity? How might you engage nonacquaintances?

_____

_____

Observation 3. What mindset can you adopt to become more comfortable in novel circumstances or environments?

_____

_____

AFFIRMATIONS:

Commitment 1. When I don't know anyone at a party, I will. . .

_____

_____

Commitment 2. I will do the following activity on my own:

_____

_____

Commitment 3. When I feel a kinship with someone I've just met, I will later reconnect with them by. . .

_____

_____

YOUR ADVICE (to revisit when you feel your circumstances need to change):

_____

_____

_____

_____

_____

ROOM TO GROW:

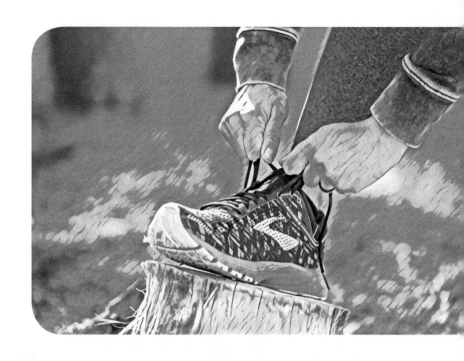

On HEALTH

I Had That Once!

Older family members will tell you their health is everything—an adage that may truly be grounded in endless progressive medical challenges. But their focus on health may also be exacerbated by loneliness, lack of purpose, and absence of something meaningful that captivates their attention. How do we attend to our health concerns while at the same time not allowing them to dominate our lives? That is the question.

MY STORY: Maybe it is just my age, but like an older car, I always seem to have something "broken." My arthritic complaints often migrate. Rotator cuff, torn hamstrings, pain in both wrists. That's not to mention more frequent headaches from any alcohol consumption, digestion concerns, and issues with my teeth and gums. What a chore! But I try to keep these issues at bay and not let them interfere with what is truly on my mind. Not easy, but if I am really focused outside of myself, it seems to work. I need to finish this book!

YOUR STORY (what **HEALTH** concerns could dominate your day?):

_____

_____

_____

_____

_____

_____

_____

_____

REFLECTIONS:

Observation 1. What can you do to direct your focus away from your health concerns?

_____

_____

Observation 2. How do you typically respond to a real health problem? For example, do you let it linger, or do you seek remedies or professional help immediately? What is the wisest choice?

_____

_____

Observation 3. Do you have a sense of what real health might feel like? What would need to change to experience that state more often?

_____

_____

AFFIRMATIONS:

Commitment 1. The next time I feel ill, I will. . .

_____

_____

Commitment 2. If I were to help someone in recovery, I would tell them. . .

_____

_____

Commitment 3. I affirm that the health of my body does not affect my spirit. To nurture my spirit, I will. . .

_____

_____

YOUR ADVICE (to revisit when you're struggling with health issues):

_____

_____

_____

_____

_____

ROOM TO GROW:

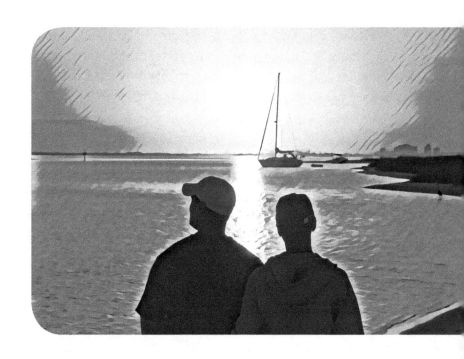

On LIGHT

Turn the Lights On

Light has an amazing effect on people. It can arouse, and it can overstimulate. It can illuminate, and it can blind. Light represents life. Without light we couldn't function. Whether it be from the sun or an irritating halogen bulb, we have to respect its power—a power that affects each of us differently.

MY STORY: When the month of May approaches, the days get longer. My seven a.m. trip to the local coffee shop is routine and something I am dedicated to throughout the year. But that trip sure is more energizing when the sun is beginning to shine through the windows. I seem more focused, my thoughts are clearer, and it is definitely more fun. I am a different guy in the light. And there is nothing like sunlight!

YOUR STORY (how does **LIGHT** affect you?):

_____

_____

_____

_____

_____

_____

_____

_____

REFLECTIONS:

Observation 1. What are the positive and negative effects that sunlight has on you?

_____

_____

Observation 2. What would your life be like without artificial light?

_____

_____

Observation 3. What does light symbolize for you?

_____

_____

AFFIRMATIONS:

Commitment 1. I will become more conscious of light because...

_____

_____

Commitment 2. When leaving a lit room, I will...

_____

_____

Commitment 3. When an older person asks whether I would like the lights on, I will...

_____

_____

YOUR ADVICE (to revisit when you're struggling to begin something new):

_____

_____

_____

_____

_____

ROOM TO GROW:

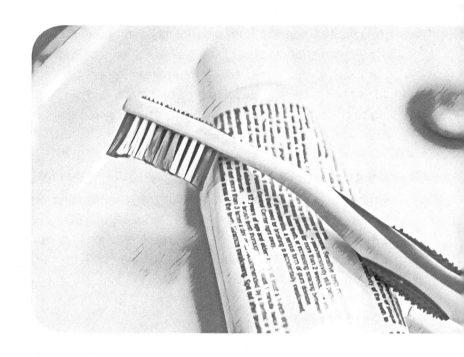

On HABITS

Decide—Today, Easy, Daily

How we structure our days significantly contributes to our success in life. Our habits, the very foundation of our lives, can work for us or against us. All positive habits—regular exercise, disciplined eating, intermittent reflection—reinforce our well-being and add to our fulfillment. But starting a new habit is challenging and may require adhering to certain ingredients for success: decide what habit you want to form, make it easy, start today, and do it daily.

MY STORY: Lately I have noticed that some of my old habits are quite secure, whereas if I attempt to start something new, I may falter. For example, in my busy day I wanted to do some brief exercises at 10:00 and 3:00. I even went so far as to create a reminder chart and put it on my desk. A practice that works most of the time. I now wonder if I am asking too much. Should I start with something easier so I'll be more motivated to practice daily?

YOUR STORY (describe a **HABIT** that you find challenging to establish):

_____

_____

_____

_____

_____

_____

_____

_____

REFLECTIONS:

Observation 1. I am very proud of the following habit I have formed:

_____

_____

Observation 2. If I could start another habit, it would be:

_____

_____

Observation 3. I know there is one thing I do that isn't good for me:

_____

_____

AFFIRMATIONS:

Commitment 1. I will decide today to start...

_____

_____

Commitment 2. To increase my chance of success, I will change my daily routine to include this good habit:

_____

_____

Commitment 3. Making the following habit easier would really help me practice it daily:

_____

_____

YOUR ADVICE (to revisit when you're not having much success forming a new habit):

_____

_____

_____

_____

_____

ROOM TO GROW:

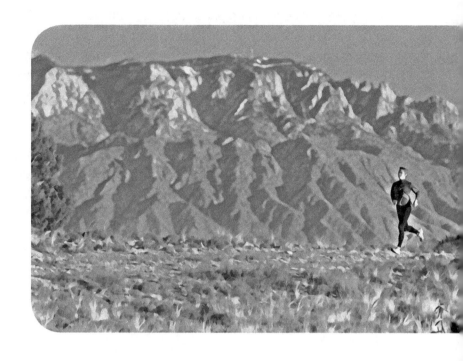

On INNER STRENGTH

Be That Person

If only life proceeded from phase to phase without a hitch. Even when we're rolling along smoothly, bumps in the road suddenly appear. And for some, life's struggles are monumental. When we are young, often our parents help to make everything better. Later, close friends come to our aid. And yet ultimately we are alone. And that is when our inner strength comes into play. Fostering our own self-reliance, whether in times of stress or during ordinary days, can be vital to living a positive and enriching life.

MY STORY: As any small-business owner knows, the height of pride in ownership is often dwarfed by the stress of business management. And few challenges rise to the level of employee issues. I am experiencing the pinnacle of such stress as I write. For reasons not inappropriate, nearly all our clinicians have resigned in recent months. The sinking feeling in the pit of my stomach has become an all-too-common feeling. Somehow I must keep going and maintain leadership of our enterprise. Fostering inner strength through personal discipline and my commitment to upholding my purpose of contributing to others' health will hopefully permit me to be the person I want to be while weathering this storm.

YOUR STORY (how has **INNER STRENGTH** helped you cope with a challenge?):

_____

_____

_____

_____

_____

_____

_____

_____

REFLECTIONS:

Observation 1. What have you learned about yourself from a moment of crisis when you felt really alone with no one to help you?

_____

_____

Observation 2. When feeling agitated, how do you calm yourself to access your inner strength?

_____

_____

Observation 3. Think of a time when you felt strong while facing difficulties. What did you do to bring out that strength?

_____

_____

AFFIRMATIONS:

Commitment 1. When under stress, I will. . .

_____

_____

Commitment 2. I will reflect on my purpose in life regularly so. . .

_____

_____

Commitment 3. When feeling overwhelmed, I will do something kind for another, such as. . .

_____

_____

YOUR ADVICE (to revisit when you're struggling with a challenge):

_____

_____

_____

_____

_____

ROOM TO GROW:

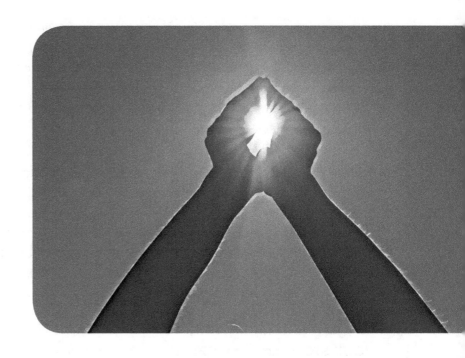

On BELIEF

Believe—or Not

We all need some constants in life: ideas, people, unwavering concepts that give us a sense of being grounded. Like habits, beliefs center us and yield a sense of security while we focus on other challenges. And beliefs facilitate decision-making. They serve as waymarks, guiding us through choices that may often seem difficult to make. And yet while beliefs provide all this, they are not immutable and can change through new experiences—for better or worse.

MY STORY: My beliefs are not centered on a spiritual practice. At times I feel wanting in this arena and have tested the waters of organized religion. Although I struggle with dogma and the concept of a higher power, I do believe in a core foundation of all religions, which is people and their desire to be good. I am ready to trust them, and with certain individuals who are close to me, securely count on them. Have I been disappointed? Yes. Some of those relationships have faltered. But I suspect that would be the case for any belief. None is perfect.

YOUR STORY how does **BELIEF** affect your life?):

_____

_____

_____

_____

_____

_____

_____

_____

REFLECTIONS:

Observation 1. What are some of your core beliefs?

_____

_____

Observation 2. What characteristics of beliefs make them meaningful to you?

_____

_____

Observation 3. Have you ever been let down by a belief? If so, how did that affect your attitude toward that belief? If not, is there anything that might shake your deeply held beliefs?

_____

_____

AFFIRMATIONS:

Commitment 1. I will be open to others' beliefs because. . .

_____

_____

Commitment 2. By taking the time to better understand my beliefs, I will. . .

_____

_____

Commitment 3. If let down by a belief, I will. . .

_____

_____

YOUR ADVICE (to revisit when you're struggling with a belief):

_____

_____

_____

_____

_____

ROOM TO GROW:

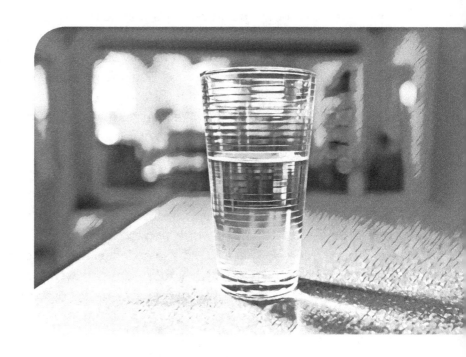

On ENOUGH

I've Had Just Enough

Often, we don't know when to stop. We want to make the dinner party perfect. We grab a snack in the checkout line at the grocery store even though we may still be full from our last meal. We just have to interview one more candidate for that position at work. We can't resist one more morsel. The positive concept of acknowledging when we've had "just enough" of something is a way to step away from it before it becomes "too much." "I've had just enough" recognizes that we generally have more than we need in life—except perhaps in the area of self-control.

MY STORY: I am nearing retirement. As a physician who has devoted a lifetime to my profession, I find ending that career to be daunting. Not only would my patients need to find another doctor who approaches cardiology the way I do, but I would lose a significant component of self-worth. And though I would be relieved of significant stress as a business owner, I would also no longer be in the game. Is there a point when I will realize my commitment to my career is over? When it has been enough? The government recognizes full retirement at age 66; baseball players when they can no longer run the bases. When is a career in cardiology enough?

YOUR STORY (describe a situation when you have had "just **ENOUGH**"):

_____

_____

_____

_____

_____

_____

_____

_____

REFLECTIONS:

Observation 1. In the situation you describe, were you successful in exhibiting self-control? What impediments went through your mind?

_____

_____

Observation 2. If unsuccessful, how might you approach the situation differently?

_____

_____

Observation 3. And if successful, how did your exercise of self-control make you feel?

_____

_____

AFFIRMATIONS:

Commitment 1. When offered dessert in a restaurant, I will consider. . .

_____

_____

Commitment 2. When shopping, I will control my urge to spend by. . .

_____

_____

Commitment 3. I will create the following boundary with people who take up too much of my time or who are in some way toxic to my well-being. . .

_____

_____

YOUR ADVICE (to revisit when you find "enough" isn't enough):

_____

_____

_____

_____

_____

ROOM TO GROW:

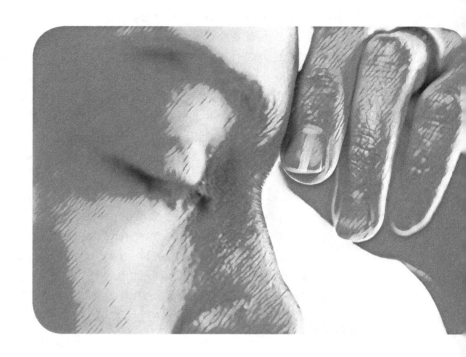

On SELF-TALK

I Did It

Each of us is responsible for our own emotional state. Optimistic and joyful, or overwhelmed and burdened. Although circumstances can influence our outlook on life, our positive attitudes must come from within. We may try self-talk as a means of emotional self-care, such as encouraging ourselves to stay the course or turn the corner. But getting behind in our emotional self-management can make the task almost insurmountable. Once negative self-talk is enthroned it is difficult to limit. When we're preparing for an upcoming situation or event, self-talk is most effective when we employ it consciously to create a positive mindset in anticipation of that situation.

MY STORY: I had to go to the dentist yesterday, not for a standard cleaning but for major oral surgery. I had undergone a similar procedure some ten years ago, but for this round I was much more apprehensive. A couple of worried nights didn't help. Driving in the car en route to the office, I had a personal pep talk: "I did it before and recovered well. The discomfort will be temporary, but above all I am a confident and forward-thinking person who will absorb this and move on." Yes, I am swollen today, but on the road to recovery!

YOUR STORY (in what circumstance have you found **SELF-TALK** helpful?):

_____

_____

_____

_____

_____

_____

_____

_____

REFLECTIONS:

Observation 1. What do you remember about that circumstance which made self-talk successful? Overall, how has self-talk worked for you?

_____

_____

Observation 2. If you haven't had an experience where self-talk has been effective for you, why do you suppose that is?

_____

_____

Observation 3. What can you do to help make self-talk more effective for you?

_____

_____

AFFIRMATIONS:

Commitment 1. I will anticipate situations in advance and prepare myself by...

_____

_____

Commitment 2. I will watch my thoughts to become aware of the kinds of negative self-talk and circular arguments I have with myself and then make a plan to...

_____

_____

Commitment 3. In practicing conscious self-talk, I will focus on creating a positive mental state of...

_____

_____

YOUR ADVICE (to revisit when you find yourself indulging in negative self-talk):

_____

_____

_____

_____

_____

ROOM TO GROW:

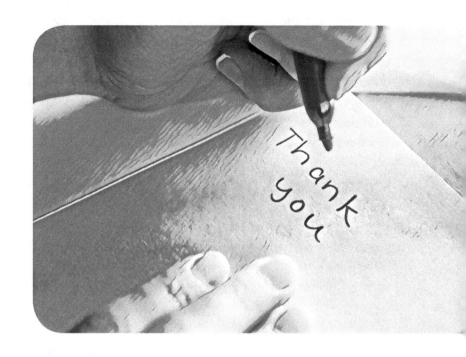

On WORDS

You Are What You Say

What we say— the words we choose—is little different from the clothes we wear. They represent us and create our brand. But being disciplined in our choice of words and the structure of our sentences is challenging. In the heat of the moment we often choose words that fail to communicate the essence of what we are attempting to say. And at times we may blunder and our choices work against us, especially when the listener interprets them far differently from what was meant. How do we ensure that our words are really us?

MY STORY: Whether to gain attention or perhaps to vent frustration, I can occasionally be acerbic in my word choices. Sharp, cutting, and critical. Maybe it creates a false sense of superiority. But the result is more often hurtful and distancing. The other day, irritated that we had run out of a supplement in our in-house pharmacy, I said to the receptionist, "What! Are we trying to create heart attacks around here?" Words that I said somewhat in jest stung the receptionist. No one came out feeling good.

YOUR STORY (pick a time you chose the wrong or perhaps the right **WORDS**):

_____

_____

_____

_____

_____

_____

_____

_____

REFLECTIONS:

Observation 1. How did the words used in your story affect the person you communicated with? How did they affect you?

_____

_____

Observation 2. Do you occasionally find yourself using words that imply criticism? In those instances, have you noticed any long-lasting effects?

_____

_____

Observation 3. A job candidate says, "Her and I went to the beach." What are your thoughts?

_____

_____

AFFIRMATIONS:

Commitment 1. In the future, if I feel critical of someone, I will. . .

_____

_____

Commitment 2. I will use words to describe ethnic groups that are. . .

_____

_____

Commitment 3. I will be careful to use proper grammar because. . .

_____

_____

YOUR ADVICE (to revisit when you find yourself being careless about your word choice):

_____

_____

_____

_____

_____

ROOM TO GROW:

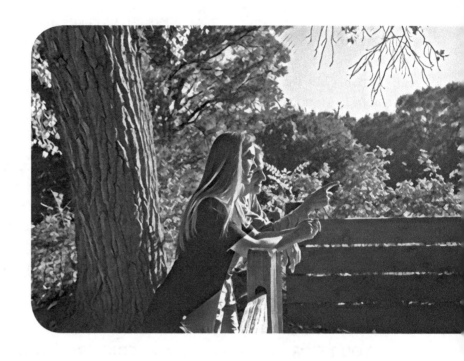

On CONVERSATION

Jump In, the Water's Warm

Engaging in conversation with strangers can be intimidating. "What will I say?" "What if I don't fit in?" "I will never see this person again." But participating in conversation, whether with friends or strangers, can be enriching—not simply because we are social creatures, but also because there can be many benefits for ourselves and others. New information, novel ways of seeing things, beneficial connections, all contribute to our growth and development.

MY STORY: We made a last-minute decision to go to the baseball game. Even though we arrived a few minutes late, we were able to purchase tickets behind home plate. Strangers sat all around us, including a seemingly nice guy in the seat to my left. A couple of innings later we struck up a conversation. Sure, some small talk: Where are you from? What kind of work? Eventually kids and photos. I reflected on what a nice guy he seemed. Ray and I are going to follow up and arrange a future health event at his office. Fortuitous.

YOUR STORY (any recent unplanned **CONVERSATIONS** that strike you?):

_____

_____

_____

_____

_____

_____

_____

_____

REFLECTIONS:

Observation 1. In what way did that conversation benefit you or perhaps the other person?

_____

_____

Observation 2. If you are comfortable initiating conversations, why do you think that's true? If not, why do you find it difficult?

_____

_____

Observation 3. Have you been in situations where you wished you had reached out to strangers? If so, what do you think you might have gained from it?

_____

_____

AFFIRMATIONS:

Commitment 1. The next time I am at a party and see some interesting people, I will...

_____

_____

Commitment 2. Engaging in conversation is important to me because....

_____

_____

Commitment 3. If someone I don't know comes up to talk with me, I will....

_____

_____

YOUR ADVICE (to revisit when you're finding it difficult to start a conversation or when you have a hard time keeping a conversation going):

_____

_____

_____

_____

_____

ROOM TO GROW:

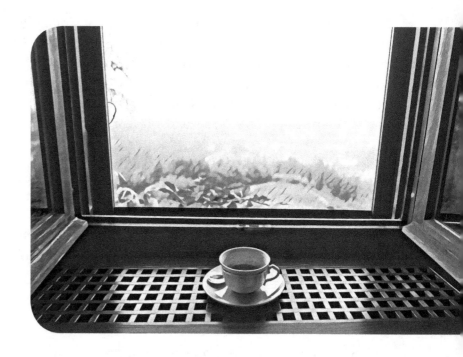

On REASONABLE

Perfection Can Be Costly

We all carry notions of the way things should be. A certain car to drive, the right wardrobe, the ideal dinner party, the spouse of our dreams. We live in a world of ideals, concepts seeded in our youth and later propagated by TV and advertising of all types. Unfortunately, we may judge ourselves by whether we have achieved some of those costly measures of outer success. Anything less is settling—and perhaps unsettling. Wouldn't it be better if the gold standard were simply what's reasonable?

MY STORY: We completed a remodel of our home about a decade ago. It was certainly not an easy job considering the state of the old ranch house. I had some dramatic ideas to open out the floor plan, raise the roof, and transcend what we had. In the end, none of those dreams came to reality, not even the granite countertops. I tell my friends that we transformed a 1960s house to a 1980s house. The outcome, though, was perfectly reasonable!

YOUR STORY (has being **REASONABLE** ever helped you adjust to reality):

_____

_____

_____

_____

_____

_____

_____

_____

REFLECTIONS:

Observation 1. How did you feel when you made that adjustment in your story? Did you feel like you were settling? Or did you accept the reality of the situation and feel at peace with your choices?

_____

_____

Observation 2. If you have a difficult time not being or having the best, what attitudes could you adopt to help you deal with this?

_____

_____

Observation 3. How might accepting what's reasonable instead of striving for perfection reduce your stress?

_____

_____

AFFIRMATIONS:

Commitment 1. I will be reasonable in future life adjustments when it comes to. . .

_____

_____

Commitment 2. The areas of my life where I will never settle are:

_____

_____

Commitment 3. When I have decided something is reasonable, I will let go and. . .

_____

_____

YOUR ADVICE (to revisit when you find yourself being unreasonable in your expectations):

_____

_____

_____

_____

_____

ROOM TO GROW:

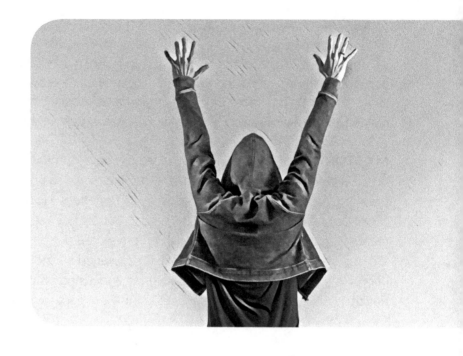

On SUCCESS

Forge On

How do we know when we arrive at success? Are we ever there? We all carry ideas of what it would mean to be successful in our lives. When we were kids, we may have hoped to follow in the footsteps of one of our parents—or certainly to be at least as successful. As we age, success becomes more complex. We set goals about having children and raising a family, getting educated and following a meaningful career, and having enough money to feel secure. Without diminishing the importance of having goals, in some instances we may never achieve complete success. But we can certainly stay inspired and keep striving.

MY STORY: Some twenty years ago I led the development of a specialty "heart hospital" in New Mexico's largest city—from brainchild to investors, design, ground-breaking, construction, and grand opening. Tremendous focus and eventual pride. The hospital was a major success. Then, to our dismay the federal government created legislation that essentially denied physicians the privilege of owning hospitals. We divested and the hospital was sold. Discouraged but not devastated, I turned my efforts to a new project—a medical enterprise focusing on preventive cardiovascular health. It's still too new to call a success, but we expect to get there!

YOUR STORY (what have you considered a **SUCCESS** in your life?):

_____

_____

_____

_____

_____

_____

_____

_____

_____

REFLECTIONS:

Observation 1. What was it about your achievement that made it a success? How did it make you feel?

_____

_____

Observation 2. What future goals can you identify that might yield a sense of success?

_____

_____

Observation 3. If you are successful at something, do you stop there? How soon after would you start something new?

_____

_____

AFFIRMATIONS:

Commitment 1. Success is personal. If pressured by others, I will...

_____

_____

Commitment 2. If I don't succeed at a goal, I will...

_____

_____

Commitment 3. Once I succeed at something, I will...

_____

_____

YOUR ADVICE (to revisit when you feel challenged by success):

_____

_____

_____

_____

_____

ROOM TO GROW:

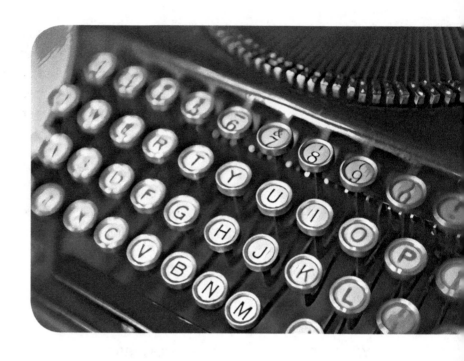

On PROGRESS

Make a Difference—Today

Progress is inevitable, and yet our relationship with progress is complex. Some progress seems to add so much benefit to our lives and to humanity. And yet some progress is deleterious—more harmful than beneficial. And as we age it becomes harder to embrace progress and all its accompanying changes. Progress we can control and design, however, is our own personal progress. What might that look like?

MY STORY: I had to replace another burned-out light bulb but couldn't find the correct wattage in our home closet. I had enough time to dash to the hardware store and knew exactly which isle to target. To my amazement, all those familiar incandescent bulbs were gone. Replaced by rows of LED bulbs. All with unfamiliar descriptors—800 lumens, just 8 watts, "bright daylight." I sure loved the glow of those old bulbs. It's a new energy-saving world. How can I embrace that more fully in my life?

YOUR STORY (an example of **PROGRESS** that is challenging for you):

_____

_____

_____

_____

_____

_____

_____

_____

REFLECTIONS:

Observation 1. Do you find progress challenging? If so, in what ways?

_____

_____

Observation 2. What emotions come to mind?

_____

_____

Observation 3. Although you may have a challenge with the progress around you, what personal progress might you make that is more in your control?

_____

_____

AFFIRMATIONS:

Commitment 1. Progress is important to humanity because. . .

_____

_____

Commitment 2. When I struggle to embrace progress, I will tell myself. . .

_____

_____

Commitment 3. I will progress in my life, and I will make a difference today by. . .

_____

_____

YOUR ADVICE (to revisit when you're struggling with inner or outer progress):

_____

_____

_____

_____

_____

ROOM TO GROW:

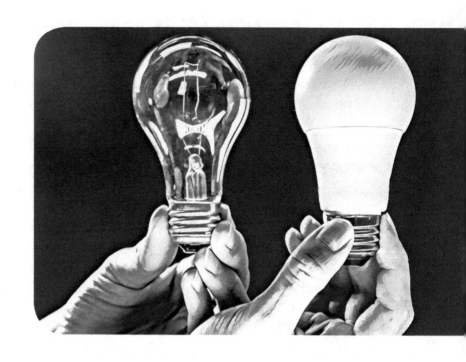

On FUTURE

Never Out of Sight

Although we are frequently reminded to live in the moment, having a keen eye to the future can be a powerful motivator in our lives. The future draws us forward, energizes us, and serves as a life propellant. And little is more effective than a strong vision of how we would like our lives to unfold—a specific career, starting a family, world travel, a new house. Whether profound or trivial, such images create anticipation and catalyze action.

MY STORY: I have had some rough going in my business lately. The medical profession is fraught with static if not declining reimbursements, and the cost of healthcare delivery is dramatically rising. These financial pressures on my business have been aggravated by significant employee turnover. Being at "retirement age," how do I stay in the fight and not simply throw in the towel. Vision! I have a vision for the future of my business that has been unwavering. Like a lighthouse guiding a ship at sea, that vision of a robust future pulls me and the business forward. Always in sight.

YOUR STORY (how has thinking of the **FUTURE** motivated you?):

_____

_____

_____

_____

_____

_____

_____

_____

REFLECTIONS:

Observation 1. How has thinking about the future and setting goals affected your life?

_____

_____

Observation 2. Do you have self-improvement goals? How might having an educational goal help you? How about clear personal health goals?

_____

_____

Observation 3. How do you adjust when your vision for the future doesn't turn out the way you expected?

_____

_____

AFFIRMATIONS:

Commitment 1. My vacation this year will be...

_____

_____

Commitment 2. I will focus on the following vision to improve my future:

_____

_____

Commitment 3. My five-year career goal is...

_____

_____

YOUR ADVICE (to revisit when the future looks bleak):

_____

_____

_____

_____

_____

ROOM TO GROW:

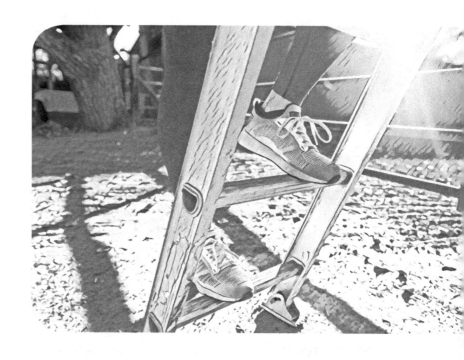

On CHORES

It's All Gotta Be Done

When has your life felt most in rhythm? When has it seemed most ordered? And when has it seemed most chaotic? Many would agree that an orderly life is built on repetitive tasks, many of which might be considered chores. Duties, obligations, must-do's. Chores, though laborious, may in fact serve a greater purpose. They can keep us humble and teach us to endure. They can also provide us with a sense of accomplishment and put us in touch with ourselves.

MY STORY: Each morning I awaken to a typical routine: shave, shower, stretch, breakfast. But the next step in my routine is different from most of my colleagues'. Rain or shine I pull on my boots and head to the barn. Cats fed, horses let out, hay for each, water troughs filled, and chickens fed. Yes, these are chores to many, and yet to me they are an important part of the start of the day. Dawn, nature, connection, out-of-doors—all returns on my daily investment.

YOUR STORY (what is your relationship to **CHORES**):

_____

_____

_____

_____

_____

_____

_____

_____

_____

REFLECTIONS:

Observation 1. Pick any common chore in your week:

_____

_____

Observation 2. Who defined the importance of that task?

_____

_____

Observation 3. Who defined the importance of that task?

_____

_____

AFFIRMATIONS:

Commitment 1. I do my chores because. . .

_____

_____

Commitment 2. In the future I will look at such tasks with. . .

_____

_____

Commitment 3. When others struggle with their chores, I will. . .

_____

_____

YOUR ADVICE (to revisit when you find yourself putting off your chores):

_____

_____

_____

_____

_____

ROOM TO GROW:

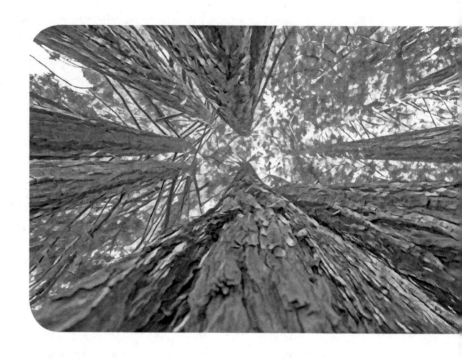

On NATURE

Look Up

We live in a remarkably artificial world: from nylon to polyester, from artificial light to near-instant heat. Countless inventions that pull us away from nature under the guise of making life easier. Are there consequences? Are we really meant to live divorced from the natural world around us? A simple pause to reflect on a time we were barefoot along a beach or alone on a forest trail may prove different.

MY STORY: A few years ago I changed my daily routine at lunch. Previously working through the lunch hour, I often felt like I was working in a submarine with little exposure to the outside world. Now I make a brief escape to our home, which is not too far from the office. With chores always to be done on our hobby farm, I spend twenty minutes cleaning the horse stalls and doing a midday animal feeding. Sounds mundane, but it puts me in contact with nature: sunshine or other weather elements, geese in the field, dirt, mud, manure—all reviving and invigorating. I'll never go back to working through lunch.

YOUR STORY (any memorable contact with **NATURE**):

_____

_____

_____

_____

_____

_____

_____

_____

REFLECTIONS:

Observation 1. Why did you choose that particular memory?

_____

_____

Observation 2. What does contact with nature do for you?

_____

_____

Observation 3. What can you do in your life to improve your connection with nature? Could it become more commonplace? If there are impediments, how can they be overcome?

_____

_____

AFFIRMATIONS:

Commitment 1. To improve my connection with nature, I will. . .

_____

_____

Commitment 2. If I find myself continually trapped indoors, I will. . .

_____

_____

Commitment 3. I will choose to live more naturally. Besides spending more time outdoors, I will. . . .

_____

_____

YOUR ADVICE (to refresh your perspective on nature when it is missing):

_____

_____

_____

_____

_____

ROOM TO GROW:

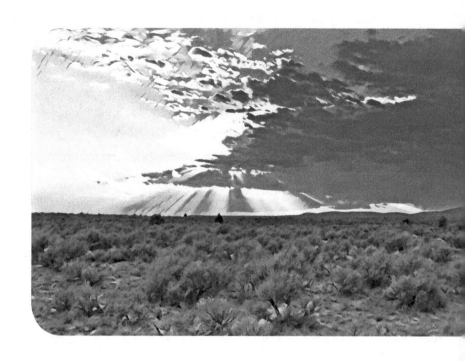

On PLACE

You Are Where You Are

Decades ago, humans were remarkably immobile. Few ventured forth. Most were born, lived, and died within miles of their parents' home. Today, even the most destitute can travel. Yet this capacity can work both for us and against us. Seeing the world is enriching, but we may often find ourselves wanting to be somewhere we are not. The place where we live both defines us as we define it. And in spite of social media, we can only be in one place at any time.

MY STORY: My family is spread throughout the world: my brother and sisters in scattered states, in-laws even farther away, wife now on the East Coast, and children equally distant. Where should I be? Home—working daily, shadowed by the dog, aloof horses, and always hungry chickens. It is easy to feel I should be elsewhere. Maybe sailing the Pacific or hiking in the Four Corners. But my profession calls. Fortunately, our office is located along the Camino Real. Flanked by the Rio Grande River, the road once connected Mexico City to Santa Fe with portions later becoming the original Route 66. Literally I do have a place. For that I must be thankful.

YOUR STORY (do you feel settled in your current **PLACE**?):

_____

_____

_____

_____

_____

_____

_____

_____

REFLECTIONS:

Observation 1. How would you describe the place where you live? Does it have meaning?

_____

_____

Observation 2. Are you invested in the place you live? If not, what could you do to become more settled?

_____

_____

Observation 3. If your location isn't optimal, how do you feel about moving to a new place? Where might that be?

_____

_____

AFFIRMATIONS:

Commitment 1. When jealous about someone who lives in another place, I will. . .

_____

_____

Commitment 2. To more fully embrace my current place, I will. . .

_____

_____

Commitment 3. When I notice that returning home feels good, I will. .

_____

_____

YOUR ADVICE (to revisit when you don't feel settled where you are):

_____

_____

_____

_____

_____

ROOM TO GROW:

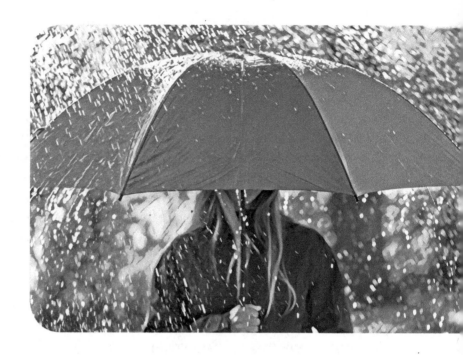

On WEATHER

Today Is Today

We are constantly enveloped in weather. Sunny, cloudy, windy, stormy, balmy. And many of us are unduly affected by our environment, including the weather of the day. Energized, discouraged, excited, calm, moody. How can we become less sensitive to the weather? How can we become less sensitive to the world around us?

MY STORY: As I woke one morning, I could hear the rain on the roof. Rain had been in the forecast, but I wasn't ready. Horses to feed, dog to let out, construction project under way. I reversed my morning routine and moved some sacks of concrete, let the riled-up horses out, and eventually called a dog with muddy feet back to the house for me to deal with, as well as the mud on my own feet! We so desperately needed the rain, but I found myself a bit irritated. I decided to have a cup of coffee and start anew. I actually had a pretty good day, and yes, the pools of water dried and the mud eventually turned to dust.

YOUR STORY (does the **WEATHER** affect you too?):

_____

_____

_____

_____

_____

_____

_____

_____

REFLECTIONS:

Observation 1. What is your favorite season? Why is it?

_____

_____

Observation 2. Would you prefer to live in a different climate? If so, why?

_____

_____

Observation 3. What do you like to do on a rainy day?

_____

_____

AFFIRMATIONS:

Commitment 1. The next time I find my mood changed by the weather, I will. . .

_____

_____

Commitment 2. If I find myself weathered by politics, I will. . .

_____

_____

Commitment 3. To better live in the moment, I will. . .

_____

_____

YOUR ADVICE (to revisit when you find yourself affected by the weather):

_____

_____

_____

_____

_____

ROOM TO GROW:

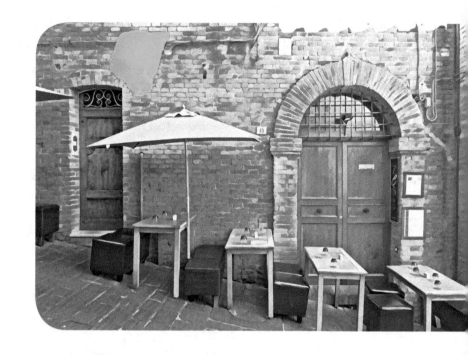

On TRAVEL

On the Road Again

On the surface, travel may seem like simple entertainment. Disneyland for kids, or a cruise on the Rhone for adults. Each an experience. Our relationship with travel is more complex. Travel often moves us out of our comfort zones. Travel creates a sense of anticipation. Travel, even the simplest, serves as a platform for personal growth. Travel energizes the self.

MY STORY: I needed to do something different for my birthday. Something meaningful, something memorable. It had been years since I had driven to one of the Indian ruins near our home. Days before, I began to make a plan. Leave early but return in time for a celebratory dinner. Pack a lunch. Take a hike? I got out several books on nearby trails and picked one along my route. Oh yes, find the camera. I went alone, which added to the impact. Six hours and two hundred miles later, I returned home. Alive!

YOUR STORY (a memorable **TRAVEL** experience):

_____

_____

_____

_____

_____

_____

_____

_____

REFLECTIONS:

Observation 1. Why did you pick that particular experience?

_____

_____

Observation 2. What emotions come to mind?

_____

_____

Observation 3. Did your travel come easily? If not, what did you do to get yourself motivated? If so, why do you suppose that is?

_____

_____

AFFIRMATIONS:

Commitment 1. The next time I'm planning to travel, I will. . .

_____

_____

Commitment 2. If I feel that the obstacles are just too many, I will tell myself. . .

_____

_____

Commitment 3. Where I go will be. . .

_____

_____

YOUR ADVICE (to remember when you're reluctant to get out of town):

_____

_____

_____

_____

_____

ROOM TO GROW:

Epilogue

Dear Journalist:

Deciding to improve your life circumstances may at times seem monumental. In picking up this Journal and embarking on its completion, you deserve great praise. I hope you found the exercise quite rewarding, not simply by taking my advice on various life challenges, but in developing your own opinions that you can both use and share with others.

Please know that I, perhaps like you, have struggled with these and similar life challenges. The answers have not come easily. Even when they do, putting them in to action is yet another challenge.

Your journey, as with all of ours, is unique. Treat it so. Bring value to each and every day and continue grow as that special person you are.

With my Best Wishes,

Dr. White (Harvey)

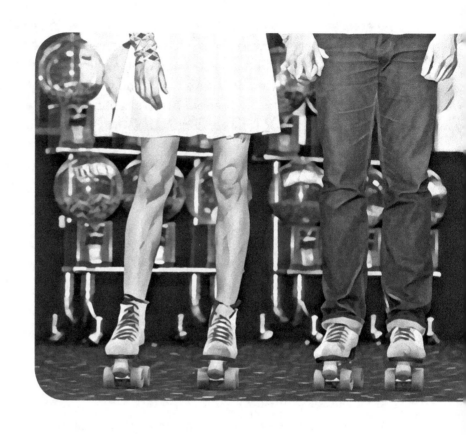

It Takes a
COMMUNITY

Acknowledgments

A career as a physician is far from static. Whether it be confronting emergencies and trauma in one's early years, or assisting older individuals to cope with their final days late in one's career, it is a pursuit of constant learning. And for having had that experience I am most grateful. Few have taught me more than my patients—some through sharing their frustrations, others with displays of pure confidence. Their stories are a constant of life lessons to be absorbed.

And as for family, I come from a long line of ministers and missionaries, whose ethos must have had some unforeseen effect on my understanding of life. For their crusade I am also grateful.

I thank my children, Martha and Haley, whose very presence, though neither would ever say it, has necessitated that I live by example, fueling an ongoing demand to do my best, to seek the most in life, and to be every bit the person I can be.

And finally, my wife, Alice, whose support has permitted my career to flourish and engender the evolution of a well-rounded professional.

* * *

This work would not have come to the page without the help and support of several individuals to whom I give great praise.

My stumbling in a search to find just the right word or phrase to express my thoughts was so helped by Santa Fean Jeff Braucher and his remarkable editing skill. He embraced every concept and assisted with enthusiasm in bringing each to print.

The layout for this journal as well as its source book was the creative effort of Diane Rigoli of Rigoli Creative (rigolicreative.com). Her energy and added vision made the graphic work stimulating, rewarding, and as much fun as writing. For all her efforts I am indebted.

Our Lifestyle Consultant at Vessel Health, Paige Kinucan, MS, was a companion throughout this adventure. Her expertise in lifestyle medicine along with her life wisdom helped in finalizing many decisions about the book and its layout. Importantly, it is her likeness that can be found in some of the accompanying photo images.

The experience of collaborating with a master photographer was also rich. The photos in this journal are the work of Kip Malone, a longtime New Mexico resident. Kip has dedicated himself to recording people's lives, institutional history, and social progress on film for the past 25 years. His engagement for this project included developing an intimate understanding of the subject matter, strategizing on photo representation, critiquing the work product, and assisting in image selection. Kip's other works can be sampled at kipmalone.com. The images included in both the On LIFE book and journal are used with his permission. I am grateful for his contribution and support.

None of this would have happened, however, without the patient guidance of Karen Bomm (iwillpublish.com). Karen devotes herself to assisting budding authors with the process of indie or independent publishing. Her years in the field and knowledge of every element of publishing shine through. She was a tireless champion of my growth as an author and provided support and encouragement throughout the experience. My indebtedness to her is without bounds.

And as Karen says: "It takes a community to build an organization, and it takes the organization's community voice to make a difference."

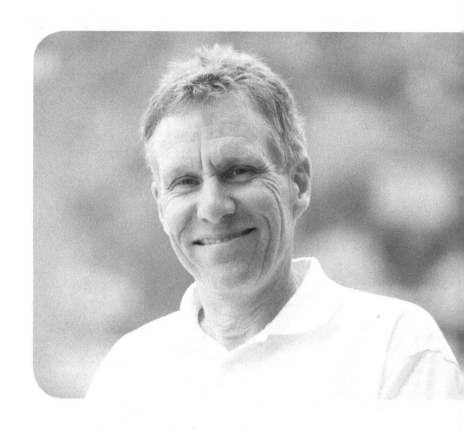

On the
AUTHOR

Harvey J. White, MD, FACC

For the past thirty-five years Dr. White has dedicated himself to direct patient care, clinical research, and leadership activities designed to improve both individual lives and our healthcare delivery system.

Building on a career in interventional cardiology, including the acute treatment of heart attack and stroke patients, Dr. White is the founder and executive director of Vessel Health, a medical enterprise pioneering prevention in the achievement of cardiovascular well-being. Former developer and medical director of the Heart Hospital of New Mexico, he has served as president of the Greater Albuquerque Medical Association, governor of the American College of Cardiology, president of the American Heart Association, and leader of the Southwest Heart Foundation.

Anchored in a profession that began as a fix-it approach for episodic health challenges, Dr. White has concluded that we, as individuals and as a society, must enhance our focus on prevention and take a proactive approach to maintaining the health of our circulatory system and promoting our personal well-being. Through Vessel Health he supports his commitment to heart health as well as to the health of the greater community. His philosophy in a nutshell: "Treat the system, not the symptom."
A career in cardiology has taught Dr. White that service as a physician entails an appreciation for the breadth of life. He has come to understand that many of our challenges are rooted in broad issues that confront us all. In this book he shares some of the observations he has developed over his years of patient care—and of simply living.

Comments and suggestions are welcome by Dr. White, who can be reached at Guide@OnLifeBook.com.

THERE IS MORE!

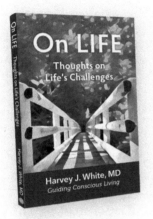

Did you know that there is a BOOK to accompany this Workbook JOURNAL?

Titled *On LIFE – Thoughts on Life's Challenges*, you will find all of the foundational concepts laid out in a simple and readable format to stimulate your thinking on the 25 topics covered in your JOURNAL. Order a copy today to add to your library!

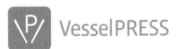

Learn more about this and other great thoughts and ideas on our website at:

VesselPressPublishing.com

Or, to learn more about Dr. White's novel preventive health business seek us out at:

Vessel Health
10601 Fourth Street NW
Albuquerque, NM 87114

505-828-3000

VesselNM.com

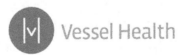

CPSIA information can be obtained
at www.ICGtesting.com
Printed in the USA
JSHW021001240321
12839JS00001B/8